THE

DIVERTICULITIS

DIET GUIDE

------------------~-----------------

A Complete Diet Guide for People with Diverticulitis

------------------~-----------------

ALSO INCLUDES: CAUSES, DIET AND OTHER REMEDIAL MEASURES

BY

MONIKA SHAH

COPYRIGHT © 2016

A Message for Readers!

Heal & Cure Diverticulitis with the Right Diet & Care

This book has been specifically designed and written for people who have been diagnosed with Diverticulitis and seriously strive to heal and cure it with the help of a right, healthy and effective homemade diet. Apart from taking medications prescribed by the doctor, it is extremely important to eat the right diet to ease the discomfort caused.

Let's take a closer look on what this book has to offer:

- **The Diverticulitis Disease Guide:** This part of the book educates, you not only about the Diverticulitis disease itself but also the causes, symptoms, risks, complications and its available treatment options in great detail. If you or any of your loved one is suffering with Diverticulitis and has to undergo the surgery, the book will educate you on the various types of surgeries available along with the post-surgery expectations and required lifestyle changes.

- **The Diverticulitis Diet Guide:** This part of the book educates you in detail about the four important and very critical stages of Diverticulitis diet that one should follow to sail through the healing period of this disease. For each of these diverticulitis diet stages, book will unfold the real goals, guidelines, diet control measures and foods to eat and avoid from various food groups in detail.

  It makes sure that the person who needs to be on diverticulitis diet is well-versed with the required dietary information and guidelines to live a healthy and painless life.

Also Includes: Natural Remedies & Self Help Measures

Apart from the Diverticulitis disease and diet guides, this book also comes with sections that will not only expand your knowledge on the various "natural remedies to cure diverticulitis" but also the critical "lifestyle changes required", once you finish through all stages of diverticulitis diet.

CONTENTS

Copyright Notes & Disclaimer

This Page Has Been Left Blank Intentionally.

Chapter 1

Understanding Diverticulitis Disease

What is Diverticulitis?

In older times, people used to have full grains, fibers and lots of vegetables. Thus, digestive diseases were rare and often unheard of. Taken into account the huge change in the consumption patterns of people around the globe in the last century, such digestive diseases have become commonplace. People have adopted diets that are high in fat and sugar content. Such diets are devoid of essential nutrients and most importantly, the fibers that help in easy digestion and effective absorption of the nutrients.

Also, people do not take care of the liquid intake in the body and consume sodas and other drinks instead of plain replenishing water. A combination of fiber deficient diet along with lack of water content in the body gives rise to conditions of constipation. People experience difficulty in passing on the stool, which gets stuck in the colon region giving rise to condition of Diverticulosis which later advances to a severe stage, called Diverticulitis.

The vegetarians are the least affected by the disease since their diet is laden with fiber coming from grains, fruits and vegetables. The non-vegetarians are at greater risk of contracting Diverticulitis. Reports have it that the meat-eating western countries like America and the European nations have greater cases of the disease than the Asian countries where several of them have a vegetarian diet as their staple food. Africans have been least affected by the disease owing to their not so rich in fat diet.

Sedentary lifestyles and lack of exercise along with proper conditioning of the body adds to the worsening of the condition. The disease is very difficult to diagnose in absence of any specific symptoms. It is often neglected in the earlier stages in lieu of ordinary digestive ailments and is not given much attention. The disease is progressive in nature and the situation deteriorates in absence of proper attentiveness.

Diverticulitis is a chronic digestive disease which involves the development of sacs or pouches in the bowel wall. These pouches are typically known as diverticula that appear on the sides of the longitudinal muscle surrounding the colon wall. This disease typically occurs in the colon or the large intestines. However, small intestines could also be affected by it.

Diverticulitis is the inflammation of one of these several diverticula. The inflammation can also be accompanied with acute infection that is often detrimental to health. Diverticulitis in its milder forms is known as Diverticulosis which is a commonly known medical condition. The most common symptoms a person with Diverticulitis shows is the excessive and continued pain in the lower abdominal region accompanied by fever and dizziness. The patient may also see sizeable increase in the white blood cell count.

The most common reason for development of the disease is assumed to be a fiber deficient diet. The disease is also associated with old age as the bowel system gets weaker as a person ages. Reports have it that almost all people above the age of 70 have been affected by Diverticulitis.

Relation between Diverticulosis and Diverticulitis

The term diverticulosis and diverticulitis are often confused with each other. People confuse themselves to have diverticulitis when all they have is common diverticulosis. Diverticulosis is a common infection while diverticulitis is a more serious condition and is caused due to acute inflammation of the bowel wall. It is not easy to cure diverticulitis and it often calls for treatment through antibiotics.

In extreme situations, patient may also be required to undergo surgery and has to be kept under prolonged medical supervision. Diverticulosis on the other hand is the condition where people have large intestinal pockets known as diverticula. This condition is sufficiently common and does pose serious consequences. It can be treated with normal dietary and lifestyle changes.

The convenient way to differentiate between the two terms is to remember the term 'itis'. Any disease ending with this term generally represents some kind of inflammation. The common medical precaution is to minimize the chances of the inflammation to burst. In case it bursts, it can be severely life threatening.

Diverticulitis is generally observed in the colon or large bowel as holes or multiple pockets. They are named as holes but have a very thin lining that prevents the stool and bacteria to pass out to the wall of the colon. The lining is excessively thin and any unwanted pressure on it causes the diverticulum to break. The breakage of this lining is responsible for the spread of bacteria and stool onto the wall of the colon thus infecting it severely. Such breakage may also lead to walled off infection that gets filled with bacteria and pus. This formation is known as abscess. The infection does not remain confined to the colon wall but is likely to spread to the other adjacent organs like ovaries, bladder, uterus etc. The bladder often suffers a condition of holes formation known as fistula. Other commonly reported situation is the passing of air while the patient urinates. Curing the abscess is a very difficult and complicated since other organs are involved and are prone to damage.

Diverticulosis has common occurrence and no significant symptoms. It is known to adopt progression and cannot be cured completely. The only way to control it is early detection and adopting preventive measures. Diverticulosis is presence of pockets in the colon which are not harmful. The real problem is the high pressured zones created due to thickened muscles known as mychosis. This thickening generates in the sigmoid colon in the left lower abdomen. This condition may cause austere narrowing and muscle buildup leading to muscle contractions. These contractions cause excruciating pain. They may also lead to extreme high pressures that can pressurize the colon walls, causing them to burst and spread infection in and around the colon wall. This is the condition which in severe cases leads to formation of diverticulitis. A high fiber diet and plentiful of liquid intake are the only ways through which diverticulosis can be kept under check.

The Causes

The causes of Diverticulitis are still under the scanner and a very clear picture of what exactly leads to the disease is a topic of debate. However, repeated studies and carefully examinations have established that intake of low fiber diet may be the major reason why the disease develops. Plenty of fiber in the diet helps to keep the stool soft and also ensures its smooth release from the body.

On the contrary, if the everyday diet is devoid of essential quantities of fiber, the stool becomes stiff and added pressure has to be applied for its release from the body. This is commonly known as the state of constipation. A low fiber diet causes formation of sacs. When pressure is applied for passing of the stool, the colon comes under undue pressure resulting in the development of diverticula.

The naturally weak places existing in the colon come under burden and result in formation of marble sized packets to protrude on the surface of the colon. This is the region where the stool gets stored before further passage. The packets do not allow the stool to completely pass and portions of it get stored in them. Diverticulitis hence occurs when faecal matter is lodged in the diverticula for extended periods of time.

Some studies also say that growth of bacteria in the packets is also responsible for the growth and inflammation in the region that surrounds the colon. The regions where the staple diet does not contain enough fiber report larger number of cases of diverticulitis. The condition of diverticulitis is commonly observed to increase with age though no substantial proof has been put forward to reinstate the fact. This however is understood and accepted since with age the bowels weaken hence increasing the possibilities of contracting the disease.

Signs and Symptoms

There are no confirmed set of symptoms that establish the presence of diverticulitis. This is why it is quite difficult to diagnose the disease particularly in the earlier stages of development. The symptoms vary from patient to patient and some cases even have patients with no prominent symptoms as such.

The most commonly observed symptom is pain in the lower region of the abdomen. The patient usually has sudden bouts of pain that are exceedingly painful. The pain has a tendency to prolong and often persists for days and even weeks in a row. Patient may experience lesser pain during certain intervals which may again aggravate to worsen the condition. Pain in the lower right side is a strong signal of presence of diverticulitis disease in the sigmoid colon.

People from the Asian descent have been commonly noted to report pain in the lower right side of their abdomen. Extreme abdominal pain understandably indicates acute perforation in the region. Apart from these, there are several other symptoms that indicate presence of diverticulitis.

- **Fever and shivering**

  If a patient is experiencing sudden fever and shivers with sensation of cold, he may be susceptible to diverticulitis.

- **Constipation and Diarrhea**

  Lack of fiber causes constipation that in the extreme case leads to diverticulitis. On the other hand, diarrhea or too frequent loose motions may also be one of the symptoms of the disease.

- **Stool stained with blood**

  If the stool excreted from the body has stains of blood over it or there is profuse or even slight bleeding from the anal opening, there is possibility that the person has diverticulitis. Constipation is the major cause of such a situation.

- **Vomiting** and **nausea** are also common symptoms.

- **Dizziness** and **continued laziness** indicate development of the disease.

- The abdomen also tends to get tender.

Risk Factors

Diverticulitis can be aggravated through certain conditions and the risk associated with it increases manifold. Proper understanding probable risks can educate susceptible patients and people in general to take preventive measures. Discussed below are some commonly understood risk factors to Diverticulitis.

- **Aging**

  Though it has not been confirmed, but age definitely has prominent relation with the impact of the disease on the human body. Growing age results in the weakening of the bowel wall. The muscular lining inside the colon and surrounding regions get fragile by the day. In extremely pressurized conditions, the colon wall is more likely to experience breakage.

People under 50 years of age are usually safe from the ill effects of the disease. People aged 60 and above are more prone to get severely affected by Diverticulitis.

- **Obesity**

  Obesity is one of the major risk factors that can lead to formation of Diverticulitis. Obesity is a direct result of improper digestion and inadequate absorption of nutrients in the body. Repeated indigestion leads to constipation that again contributes to development of Diverticulitis.

  Even in the case where the patient has been diagnosed with disease, obesity can cause hindrance in proper treatment especially in the cases where surgeries are inevitable. Excess layers of fat make it difficult to penetrate to the affected areas in the interior regions of the body. Consequently, the healing is slower and extended medical supervision becomes obligatory.

- **Smoking**

  Though a detailed reasoning is unavailable, regular smokers are at greater risk of contracting the disease than non-smokers.

- **Excessive consumption of animal fat**

  Animal fat, particularly red meat is very high in fat content. Regular intake of diet rich in animal fat is not desirable in the long run. It increases the cholesterol levels in the body, triggers obesity and is a major cause of constipation and persistent indigestion. People solely dependent on a meaty diet are more likely to suffer from Diverticulitis.

- **Fiber deficient diet**

  Again, a fiber deficient diet will escalate the progression of Diverticulitis at a much faster pace.

- **Insufficient intake of fluids**

  People who forget to maintain proper fluid levels in their body often complain of constipation. As discussed earlier, constipation will lead to higher possibilities of contracting Diverticulitis.

- **Lack of exercise**

  Each of the risk discussed above boils down to the one simple yet critical risk associated with lack of exercise and physical activity. Sedentary lifestyle and improper attention to health makes the body weak and prone to acquiring diseases. The worst affected by this is the digestive system which is at the core of entire well-being of the human body.

- **Medications and treatments**

  There are several medications that may elevate the risk of Diverticulitis. This could either be a side effect or a direct impact of use of those medications. The common names under such medications are opiates, steroids and non-steroidal anti-inflammatory drugs like Naproxen and Ibuprofen.

These are some of the widely observed risks that may advance propagation of Diverticulitis in the human body.

This Page Has Been Left Blank Intentionally.

Chapter 2

Diverticulitis Complications

Abscess

The abscess is the most common type of complication that arises because of Diverticulitis. It is in the form of a small protruding ulcer that develops on the outer surface of the large intestine. It is like a fissure that is filled with liquid pus. It can also be in form of a lump in the tissue. The very widely used technique used for correcting the abscess is known as PAD defined as Percutaneous Abscess Drainage.

The exact location of the abscess is located by the use of a CT scan. A tube like instrument connected with a needle is inserted in the body through the abdomen. The needle is used to drain out the pus from the abscess. For this entire PAD process, local anesthesia is utilized. The process might need to be repeated in case the size of abscess is really large. Antibiotics alone can be used for the drainage of the pus where the size of the abscess is less than 1.5 inches.

Perforation

Perforation occurs in severe cases where the infected diverticulum commonly called a pouch suffers breakage. This breakage leads to the spreading of the infection in the lining surrounding the abdomen. This spreading of infection is medically termed as peritonitis.

This condition develops in extremely severe cases that are neglected for elongated periods of time. It is quite possible that the patient may develop threat to his life. Immediate cure is required here with use of antibiotics. In case where the condition is really out of control, surgery is used to remove the pus from the affected region. A process called colostomy is also put to use to direct the large intestine towards the abdomen for better treatment.

Peritonitis

As discussed above peritonitis is the spreading of infection in and around the abdominal lining. The infection in the abdominal lining causes inflammation in the area. This area is known is peritoneum. This type of infection is very likely to spread quickly in the entire body. Hence, it is very important to take instant measures to bring medical assistance to the patient. The condition of peritonitis is characterized by the presence of high fever and a very severe abdominal pain that becomes unbearable after a certain point. The patient experiences a sudden drop in his appetite and the urination patterns also alter. In fact they suddenly drop or the patient in some cases does not urinate at all. The treatment is mostly done through antifungal medicines and in some cases even antibiotics. Surgery is the only option that remains in very severe cases.

Rectal Bleeding

Statistics have it that around 20% percent people inflicted by diverticulitis may experience some form of bleeding. This bleeding is not painful at all. It lasts for a very small duration. It is known to cure by itself and does not really pose big threat to life. However, you are in need of medical attention if the bleeding is profuse and does not stop by itself. Excessive bleeding may also call for blood transfusion to make up for loss of lost blood from the body. It is strongly advised to seek medical monitoring in case of excessive bleeding or it may worsen due to delay.

Fistula

A fistula is another very commonly observed complication caused by diverticulitis. Fistulas are unusual openings that connect together the different parts of the body. These hence also connect the tissues of the abdominal lining and the intestine together. The infected tissues have the tendency to stick together with each other. Upon recovery of the tissues there is possibility of formation of a fistula. This formation can cause the transfer of infection from the large intestines to other parts of the body. For example the bladder is one organ that can get severely infected by this. Surgery is the common way to remove the infected part the colon that contains the fistula.

Intestinal Obstruction

It is possible that the infection spreads too much to cause damage and subsequent blockage of the large intestine. This blockage needs immediate medical supervision in absence of which the large intestine will start to fall apart and decay. This will create breeding grounds for peritonitis.

If the large intestine is partially blocked, it may still not be as threatening. But it will surely affect the patient's ability to digest food and absorb nutrients. The patient may also experience excruciating pain.

Intestinal obstruction is rarely observed to be caused by diverticulitis. Cancer is supposedly a bigger cause for this. The reason for intestinal obstruction can be established only after careful examination of a seasoned medical practitioner. The most widely used way to remove the blockage is surgery. In critical situations, colostomy is also used which can be temporary or permanent, depending on the situation. Untreated blockages may result in serious and prolonged problems with digestion.

Chapter 3

Diverticulitis Treatment Options

Diverticulitis may exist in acute or severe forms. Each of these forms poses a complicated or uncomplicated situation. Depending on the severity of the situation, a particular method is adopted for the treatment of diverticulitis. Most of the patients suffering from acute form of uncomplicated disease have been known to be cured using antibiotics. For complicated cases, surgery is the way to follow which may improve the condition.

Diet

Diverticulitis is a direct result of a fiber deficient diet. Foods rich in fats like red meat and excessive refined flours are responsible for causing conditions of indigestion and constipation. Those people who refrain from taking adequate intakes of fiber from fruits and vegetables also slowly invite the risk of developing diverticulitis. In the initial stages when the disease is detected, it is possible to cure the disease by making alterations in the diet. It is strongly advised that the patient should opt for liquid diet that is easy to digest.

Along with a liquid diet, a combination of low fiber foods is also included in the diet. When detected early, most cases of diverticulitis can be cured with proper diet and a combination of few antibiotics.

Antibiotics

Antibiotics are the first adopted method to cure diverticulitis. If the condition is well diagnosed in the earlier stages itself, the treatment can be controlled with the use of antibiotics only making the need of surgery unnecessary. In cases of uncomplicated diverticulitis, treatments can also be done at home with the right prescription of medicines.

Antibiotics restrict the spread of the infection. Accompanied with a liquid diet for a few days, the affected area in the bowel will get healed slowly and steadily. It is possible to add solid food to your diet once the symptoms slowly start to diminish. This method is known to successfully cure about almost everyone with uncomplicated diverticulitis.

In case of complicated diverticulitis, the antibiotics are sufficiently strong in their action and at many times need to be directly injected into the patient's body. In some cases, needles are injected with the help of tubes to suck out the pus from the blisters formed in the form of abscess.

CT Scan-Guided Percutaneous Drainage

It is not always that a patient will respond positively to the doses of antibiotics. Sometimes significant CT scans reveal presence of prominent abscess in the colon. If registered early, the pus from the abscess can be drained out without the need of the surgery and most undesirable state where colostomy needs to be administered.

Guided Percutaneous drainage is the method to remove the abscess in early stages. PAD also makes use of intravenous application of antibiotics. This is known to look at two major aspects. First is the primary sepsis treatment and the second is the curing of sigmoidectomy that has been characterized by the radical improvements in the treatments done through radiology and the ability of CT scans to locate important locations of the abscess formation.

CT scan procedure may include antibiotic application through intravenous, oral or rectal methods. A small needle is inserted in the skin leading to the location of the identified abscess. The pus is then drained out of the abscess. The patient is mostly hospitalized. The situation is more identifiable using CT scan in case where patients have Hinchey Stage II diverticulitis. This procedure helps the patient to heal faster than any kinds of surgical treatment used to operate the abscess.

Surgery

Diverticulitis may cause worsened conditions where a surgery is inevitable. The conditions where the patient develops bowel obstruction, fistula or prominent abscess are the times where the doctors resort to surgery. In case where minor symptoms of diverticulitis persist or there is repeated occurrence of uncomplicated type of diverticulitis, a severe situation may develop.

Immediate surgery is required where the patient has really large abscess and incurs profuse bleeding accompanied by clear symptoms of peritonitis. A weak immune system and low body resistance combined with an inability to digest certain foods can result in the more profound and complicated stages of diverticulitis.

The surgical treatment is undertaken using two procedures which are discussed as follows:

- The first surgery is where the doctor applies cleaning agents to clear off the affected surface in the abdomen. He then operates the region and gets rid of the portion in the colon affected by the abscess. A temporary colostomy is then exercised to create an opening or passage in the abdomen. The medical fraternity commonly defines this opening as stoma. This opening is created with the view to attach the end of the colon with the stoma. This makes it feasible for the patient to continue with his normal eating routine while the wound undergoes healing.

  A pouch like mechanism is attached to the end of the opening where the stool gets deposited. Hence, the patient continues to heal while the body continues with its everyday processes. This type of surgical treatment is medically known as primary bowel resection.

- In some extreme cases, it is not possible to correct the situation using the surgical procedure described above. The inflammation is beyond control and that is where surfaces the inability for the surgeons to join the ends of colon with that of the rectum. This can be only done with the use of colostomy. A stoma is again created on the surface of the abdomen and a fresh, unaffected and healthy part of colon is then attached to it. The wastes are again excreted out using the opening and the wound continues to heal. The wound is then observed until the inflammation goes down.

If the situation allows, the colostomy process can be put on reverse mode and bowel may be reconnected to its original position rendering perfect placements of the abdominal body organs. This means that the ends of the colon are rejoined with each other while the stoma is closed eventually.

Risks of Surgery

The surgery for diverticulitis is an expensive affair, especially if there is an immediate need for colostomy. The risk of surgery is quite high since diverticulitis is a form of inflammatory disease. This inflammatory nature of the ailment calls for extensive care while operating the affected region of the colon.

The risks involved with diverticulitis do not develop overnight since growth of the disease is slow and incremental and if noticed early, most risks can be eliminated to a state where no surgery is required.

Few repercussions of the surgeries can be the following:

- **Acquiring Infections**

  After the surgery, there is a pronounced risk of acquiring some kind of infection since surgeries open up the body organs and make them more prone to acquiring infections. It is very important to cleanse the wound regularly and sterilize it and cover it with a bandage. It is normal to have some redness around the wound but profuse yellowish or transparent discharge from the wound indicates the presence of infection that needs instant medical attention.

- **Diarrhea and Nausea**

  A patient is very likely to feel nauseated after the diverticulitis surgery. A low fiber and easily digestible diet is the major requirement in such a situation. The shortening of the colon causes the stool to get ejected faster thus causing diarrhea. Diet is the only way these conditions can be controlled.

- **Fever**

  There is a risk of developing acute fever after the surgery. Sometimes the fever tends to go beyond the acceptable limits causing shivers and chills. It is advisable to rush the patient to the doctor in such a condition.

- **Constipation**

  A low fiber diet needed for recovery will again cause constipation for the patient. This is a risk to the patient since the wound is still recovering and if constipation arises again, it may cause opening of the wounds and delay in the healing process.

What to Expect After the Surgery

The time succeeding the operation will be a crucial one wherein proper care and rest will determine the pace of the recovery. A general anesthesia is generally employed for the resection of the bowel. The patient is generally kept under medical supervision for about a week that may extend up to a period of about 15-17days.

The formation of stoma is for the purpose of allowing the faecal matter to pass out from the body through the process of colostomy.

In the case where double surgery is required, the difference between the surgeries is around 5 to 11 weeks. The general recovery time is a month to two months. However, the recovery time also varies depending on the health and age of the patient as well as the kind of treatment the patient has undergone. The conventional surgery usually takes longer to heal while the ones using laparoscopic procedure usually heal faster.

Post the surgery, all the nutrition and medication is fed through intravenous procedures. The generally observed procedure is to drop in a tube through the nasal cavity leading to the stomach through which liquid food is passed into the patient's system. This however is used only for a few days. The patient is slowly brought onto a liquid diet and the intravenous mechanism is removed.

If the patient is able to pass on the gas from the system, the patient is administered to a liquid diet. Passing of the gas is a clear indication of the healing of the colon. The case where a person is comfortably able to take up liquid diet without experiencing any kind of pain in the abdominal region, some form of semi-solid foods can also be incorporated in the diet.

Since the body is still damaged and is in state of repair, the patient is kept on a diet that is particularly low in fiber. The diet will continue to benefit within at least a period of 15 days to 2 months. The simple reason behind a low fiber diet is the ease of digestion owing to which the wound will be able to heal faster. All care needs to be taken to avoid strenuous work since the abdominal region is still weak.

It is necessary to take complete rest though little activity is advisable. Again, if a patient undergoes normal surgery, recovery will be prolonged while in case of laparoscopic procedure, the recovery is relatively faster and it is quicker for the patient to resume the daily activities of life.

After Discharge Expectations and Guidelines

As discussed above, a patient should not expect sudden improvement in the condition after the surgery. Diverticulitis surgery is a sensitive surgery that requires time and patience to heal. Adequate rest is strongly advised with no strenuous movements. A low fiber diet will be commonplace in the patient's lifestyle for quite some time until he does not complain of any acute pain in the abdomen.

The following are the common guidelines that doctors prescribe post the surgery for treatment of diverticulitis:

- The patient should undergo sufficient rest for about 30 days to two months depending on the kind of treatment.

- The diet should be low on residue as well as in fiber thus enabling easier digestion and healing of the wounds.

- Proper cleansing of the wound is crucial and if any infection develops, immediate medical attention should be provided.

- Regular check-ups are advised for doctors to monitor the rate and extent of healing.

- The diet should be changed gradually and the solids should be incremental incorporated slowly after carefully assessing the state of the wound and how the patient is responding to the medications post-surgery.

- It is also necessary to carefully monitor the passages or openings from where the wastes from the body are removed since there is a very high possibility of spread of infection even from that area.

This Page Has Been Left Blank Intentionally.

Chapter 4

The Diet Guide for Diverticulitis

Again and again the importance of diet is being restated for the treatment of diverticulitis. Diet alone can be the sole reason because of which the body recovers out of acute and severe conditions of the diverticulitis disease. In cases of early diagnosis, when the condition is still better and only diverticulosis has come into picture, diet is the very common and effective way that can make the disease sure faster and better.

It is advised to adopt a fiber rich diet throughout the lifetime to reduce the risk of contracting the disease especially in the older age. During treatment varieties of diet are incorporated at different stages that mostly include fruits, vegetables, roughage and lots of fiber along with plentiful fluids and water as a major component. More than the reduced complexity of the food that is being adopted, it is the willingness to stick to these diets consistently, that will protect against the disease.

These diet and diet foods are fairly simple in nature and can be found easily in the households. One rule goes without saying, the simpler the better! Most of these diets are inspired by the simple eating patterns of the primitive age where emphasis was on a fiber rich diet accompanied by whole grain foods that are very easy to digest. Here's a look at an extensive diet guide to combat diverticulitis disease.

Stage 1: The Clear Liquid Diet

A clear liquid diet for the treatment of diverticulitis is advised post-surgery or a stage exceeding acute complicated diverticulitis. Post-surgery, the abdominal region, particularly the intestinal region and any area that has been operated in and around the colon experience a strong meltdown in their ability to function. This slowdown in bodily functions and the existing wounds make it difficult for them to digest food and process it as they normally do. Any added pressure on these areas because of any kinds of heavy foods may cause outbreak of infection and lead to persistence of the condition.

Goals

The following are the goals of adhering to a clear liquid diet:

- **Giving proper rest to the intestinal region**

  By intake of cleared liquid foods, the abdomen is saved of so much of stress. The digestion becomes quicker and smoother. This allows the intestine to be at rest while the operated region steps back to its original functioning.

- **Strengthen the intestines for digestion**

  Clear liquid diet act as cleansers that wash of the abdominal and intestinal region of any undesired bacteria and enzymes that are causing the condition to persist. Regular intake of clear liquid diets will flush off all the toxicities and create a healing environment more acceptable to nutrition intake.

- **Easy excretion**

  After the diverticulitis surgery, the colon and rectum are usually in bad shape. The pouches in the colon are still in recovery mode and hence passing of the stool becomes a problem. A clear liquid diet ensures passing of excreta in most painless way possible. Since most of it is liquid part and contains water, a substantial amount of excretion occurs through urination which is mostly effortless. And hence protects the patient from further damage.

- **Maintenance of hydration**

  Most surgical treatments rely on heavy antibiotics post treatment. These drain the hydration out of the body making it highly deficient in water content. One of the aims of liquid diets, is to replenish the body of all the lost water content. Along with the water content, such diets also replenish the electrolyte and vitamin levels in the body bringing back sodium, potassium levels to the required levels.

Clear liquid diets also improve overall body health particularly targeting the gut region that may be prone to leaky gut syndrome. The cellulite levels may also be reduced significantly. All of this eventually helps the digestive tract to heal faster and function better.

Guidelines for Clear Liquid Diet

The following are the guidelines to be followed while making clear liquid diets for the cure of diverticulitis:

- Clear liquid diets have to be necessarily liquid foods. The commonly accepted norm is that any natural food that remains liquid at the room temperature can be considered for liquid diet.

- Clear liquid diets are based solely on liquids. They may replenish electrolyte and vitamin levels to certain extent, but they still lack in essential components like carbohydrates and proteins. Lack of these essential components can make the body weak and prone to other diseases and ailments. Hence, a liquid diet should never be prolonged. It is best to seek medical prescription before undertaking a clear liquid diet. Ideally it should continue for 5-7 days.

- No kind of solids should be included in a clear liquid diet which necessarily has to be liquid.

- Clear liquid diets can be hard to stick onto. They can be repetitive and uninteresting. However, this problem can be solved by making using of variety of colorful ingredients that can be used to make juices, broths and soups. This will make the diet easier to follow and the patient will recover sooner. The cleansing action of the clear liquid diet increases appetite by improving digestion.

Foods to Include & Exclude in Clear Liquid Diet

The following foods should be included in a clear liquid diet:

- Plenty of water whether plain, flavored or carbonated will keep the hydration levels in check.

- Tea and coffee without added milk sugar or cream can be used as liquid diet. Too much this can however lead to dehydration.

- Fruit juices of all kinds especially those of oranges, apples, pineapples etc. can be used as liquid foods. The pulp should not be included as it classifies under semi-solid foods.

- Juices of vegetables especially tomato can be of great help.

- Lemonades and punches with a pinch of honey and sugar make up for great liquid diets.

- Broths are another great way to have clear liquid diets. Vegetable broths are desirable. Non-vegetarians can opt for chicken broths and fish soups. All of these are appreciably nutritious and appetizing.

- Ice pops are popular clear liquid diet but should be taken without any nuts or milk.

- Gelatin intake is also advised in most cases.

What to Avoid?

Avoid any kinds of solid and semi-solid foods. Apart from the ones mentioned above, most foods should be avoided. Intestine and gut are sensitive to certain kinds of food hence an allergic test is advised before going on any kind of clear liquid diet.

Stage 2: The Juicing Diet

After the completion of a certain days of clear liquid diet, the affected patient can be put on a diet of fruit and vegetable juices. This is one step up when a patient shows significant improvement. It is required that organic fruits and vegetables are used in these conditions since their benefits rank higher for obvious reasons.

Goals

The goals of a juicing diet are as follows:

- Juicing diets are incorporated to mark slow transition of a diverticulitis patient from early post-surgery stages to a more stable state where the digestion has considerably improved.

- They are used to make the body adaptable to increased amounts of nutrients and vitamins.

- Juicing diets also complement the high dosage of antibiotics and make them more effective.

- Juicing diets are aimed at bringing back the lost nutrition from the body that has been lost over a period of time.

Guidelines for Juicing Diet

- The juicing diet should be started only when significant improvement has been shown in the patient's condition.

- It is desirable to use organic fruits and vegetables to facilitate the best healing conditions.

- The fruits and vegetables should be well strained and should be clear of any kinds of seeds, fibers or skin. In this case, any food with high amount of seeds or a tough skin should be completely avoided. There is a very chance of these seeds, fiber and skin to get accumulated in the sacs created by the diverticulitis disease in the colon and the intestinal region. Once, they get stuck, it is very difficult to get them out. Not only will they be difficult to remove, they will delay or block the healing of the operated pouches.

- Juices of different fruits and vegetables should be given to the patient from time to time to include variety of nutrients in the diet. Making seedless thin pulp of the fruits and vegetables is also a popular way to stick to the juicing diet. This pulp will be digestive and will be instrumental in further cleaning of the duct.

Fruits to Include & Exclude in a Juicing Diet

Here is an elaborate list of fruits to be included and excluded in a juicing diet.

Fruits to be included:

- Apples juice is very rich in anti-oxidants and very digestive in nature.

- Cherries of different kinds, peaches, grapes, oranges, prunes are the best kinds of fruits to be juiced for the cure of the diverticulitis disease.

- However, one has to make sure that too acidic juices are not to be taken in large quantities since they may cause eruption of the interior of the intestinal skin.

Fruits to be excluded:

As mentioned previously, any fruit with really hard texture, skin or too many seeds should not be included in the juicing diet. Guavas for example are stiff in texture and also contain too many seeds. They are clearly unsuitable as an option for diverticulitis juicing diet.

Vegetables to Include & Exclude in a Juicing Diet

Vegetables to be included:

- The same rule also goes in for vegetables as the fruits. Look for soft and juicy vegetables that are sans to many seeds. Tomatoes are the best option since they can be used for making different kinds soups, juices, broths etc. It is easy to blend tomatoes with other vegetables to make juices that are appealing, healthy and appetizing.

- Green leafy vegetables like watercress, lettuce and spinach can be used to make vegetable juices that alleviate the condition of the patients affected by diverticulitis disease.

Vegetables to be excluded:

Diverticulitis is characterized by presence of pouches or sacs in the intestine. Hence, all vegetables with seeds, skins and excess fiber needs to completely eliminated from the diet. All the vegetables that cause gas in the stomach should be kept away. These vegetables stimulate the digestive tract too much causing discrepancies. These vegetables include carrots, beans, even beat root. Kale is again a leafy vegetable but is supposedly too fibrous and causes gas. Hence, even this should be avoided.

Stage 3: The Low Residue Diet

Once the intestinal healing has processed, liquid diets can be furthered to low residual diets that bring in some kind of fiber into the diet. The term "**Residue**" refers to the indigestible content of food we eat. Foods that contain a residue increase the stool weight and the fecal residue. Such foods are therefore to be avoided if you need to be on a low residue diet. Foods that are high in residue include high fiber foods like fruits and vegetables. You may also need to avoid tough and fibrous meats with gristle (an animal tissue that is difficult to digest) as they add to more residues and hence must be avoided.

A low residue diet contains foods that are very easy to digest, pass and do not cause a blockage. On a low residue diet it is important to avoid foods that are high in fiber content. The term "**Fiber**" refers to the portion of carbohydrates (starch) that humans cannot digest. Fiber passes through the digestive tract mostly unchanged and hence not recommended during low residue diet.

Goals

- The major goal of a low residue diet is to establish acceptance for fiber in the body. The key is to start slowly and not bombard the body with top much of fiber intake in the midst of the healing process.

- A low residual diet will be certainly rich in nutrients than the clear diet and the juicing diet. Thus, one of the goals of the low residual diet is to improve the quality of nutrients being fed to the body.

Guidelines

The key to switching to a low residue diet is to include easily digestible low fiber foods. The fiber content should be enough to trigger improved digestion. This can be achieved using unprocessed grains and whole foods and starches. The fruits and vegetables should also be used in their raw form as and when possible. Slight processing is also acceptable as long as the fiber and nutrient stay in place.

Basic Principles of a Low Residue Diet

There are some basic principles of low residue diet that one should always follow. These are in addition to the foods that should not be consumed during the course of a low residue diet. Let's take a quick look at these principles:

- A low fiber diet must not contain more than 10-15 grams of fiber per day.

- Foods with some fiber like fruits and vegetable must be well cooked.

- Avoid highly seasoned foods. It is not required to completely stop seasoning the food.

- You just need to make sure that the food is seasoned in moderation.

- Avoid eating large meals as they may cause discomfort from gastric distention.

- Avoid frying completely and try to cook by baking, boiling, broiling, roasting, stewing, microwaving, or creaming.

Foods to Include & Exclude in Low Residue Diet

Unlike other diet programs, low residue diet offers a wide variety of foods that can be consumed. In this chapter you will be able to identify the list of foods from various food groups that should be included to and avoided from a low residue diet program. Let's have a look at these foods and food groups in detail.

Breads and Starches

Breads and starches are the most significant sources of carbohydrates that have been lost in a body recovering of diverticulitis. It is to be noted that low residue diets should focus on brown breads with soft crusts. Even white breads can be included in decent quantities. Starches from potatoes, rice and pastas can be included in the diet.

It has to be made sure that at this stage, no coarse and whole grains should be a part of the diet. Nut, dry fruits and seeds are to be completely avoided since they have a hard skin and are also coarse. The following is a list of allowed and not allowed foods for Breads and Starches food group.

Allowed Foods	Foods to Avoid
- White breads	- Wholemeal bread and flour
- Muffins	- Granary bread and flour
- Rolls	- Wholemeal pasta
- Biscuits	- Quinoa

- Crackers	- Pearl barley
- Light rye bread (seedless)	- Brown rice
- Pancakes	- All cereals that contain whole wheat
- Waffles	- Muesli
- Corn flakes	- Porridge
- Special k	- All foods that contain nuts and dried fruits
- Rice krispies	
- Puffed rice	
- White potatoes	
- Sweet potatoes (without skin)	
- White rice	
- Pasta	
Refined cooked cereals like:	
- Cream of rice	
- Cream of wheat	
- Farina	
- Grits	

Note: Products that are made with coconut, nuts, bran, seeds or dried fruits are very high in fiber and leave a great amount of residue and hence not recommended in this diet.

Meat and Protein

Tender meats like those of fish, eggs, peanut butter (without bits) and cottage cheese and yogurt are excellent sources of protein for the treatment of diverticulitis. The following is a list of allowed and not allowed foods for Meat and Protein food group.

Allowed Foods	Foods to Avoid
- Ground, tender or well cooked meats	- Tough and gristly meat
- Poultry	- Skin and bones of fish
- Tofu	- Pies containing vegetables
- Fish	- Egg dishes containing vegetables (as listed in the allowed vegetables section, later in this chapter)
- Eggs	
- Creamy peanut butter	**Legumes (peas and beans)**
	- Kidney beans
	- Lima beans
	- Navy beans
	- Black beans
	- Soy beans
	- Split black eyed beans
	- Chickpeas
	- Garbanzo
	- Pinto beans
	- Peanuts
	- Yellow peas
	- Lentils
	- Crunchy peanut butter

Vegetables

One has to particularly stick to soft leafy vegetables that are not very fibrous. Pumpkin, tomato juice, mushroom soup, strained beat root juice will escalate the healing process. Avoid mostly all kinds of hard textured vegetables like whole beat root, turnips, carrots, radish etc. The following is a list of allowed and not allowed foods for Vegetables food group.

Allowed Foods	Foods to Avoid
- Cucumber	- Raw vegetables and salads
- Green pepper	- Split peas
- Romaine	- Lentils
- Tomatoes	- Peas
- Onions	- Sweet corn
- Zucchini	- Celery
	- All seeds
	- All pips
	- All tough skins
	- Potato skins
	- Baked beans
	- Lima beans
	- Green peas
	- Broccoli
	- Parsnips
	- All others
	- Juices with pulp or bits

Note: **All vegetables are allowed except the ones that are not recommended.**

Fruits

All types of soft fresh and canned fruits can be included in the diet. All other kinds of fruits should be avoided. The following is a list of allowed and not allowed foods for Fruits food group.

Allowed Foods	Foods to Avoid
- Apricot	- All dried fruits
- Peach	- Citrus fruit

- Plum	
- Honeydew	**Berries**
- Nectarine	- Strawberries
- Papaya	- Blackberries
- Banana	- Raspberries
- Cantaloupe	
- Watermelon	- Prunes
- All juices without pulp and strained	- All Smoothies
	- Fruit juices with bits

Note: **All fruits are allowed except the ones that are not recommended or those with seeds or skins.**

Dairy Products

Yogurt is highly recommended at this stage. Milk, milk shakes and soft smoothies can be included in the low residue. Even cottage cheese is favorable. All other kinds of dairy product are to be avoided. The following is a list of allowed and not allowed foods for Dairy food group.

Allowed Foods	Foods to Avoid
- Yogurt	- Products with seeds and nuts in them
- Cheese	
- Milk	

Fats

Light fats are to be used in a low residue diet. Any kind of butter, vegetable oil, cream and margarine can be used. Only heavy oils and salad dressings especially those made from olive oil are to be excluded. The following is a list of allowed and not allowed foods for Fats food group.

Allowed Foods	Foods to Avoid
- Butter	- Nuts
- Bacon	- Seeds
- Salad dressings	- Coconut
- Vegetable oils	- Olives
- Mayonnaise	- Poppy seed dressings
- Margarine	- Crunchy peanut butter
- Cream	
- Whip cream	
- Plain gravies	
- Creamy peanut butter	

Sweets and Desserts

Highly processed sweets and desserts are to be avoided at this stage. Sweetness quotient can be added to the diet using honey, sugar and fruit jellies. Do not consume dried nuts, fruits or coconut dishes. The following is a list of allowed and not allowed foods for Sweets and Deserts food group.

Allowed Foods	Foods to Avoid
- Pastries	Any product(s) that is made using or contain(s) the following:

- Pies	- Whole grains
- Sugar	- Bran
- Plain hard candy	- Coconut
- Condiments	- Nuts
- Coffee	- Seeds
- Tea	- Dried fruits
- Carbonated beverages	- Chocolate syrup
- Sherbet	- Candies made with chocolates or nuts
- Gelatine	- Horseradish
- Sponge cakes (without fruit and nuts)	
- Jelly	**More Foods to Avoid**
- Ice cream	- Cakes, puddings and biscuits made using wholemeal flour, nuts and dried fruits
- Custard	- Chocolate with dried fruit or nuts
- Semolina and rice puddings	- Toffees with dried fruit or nuts
- Jams without seeds	- Fudge with dried fruit or nuts
- Plain biscuits	- Marmalade with peel
	- Jams with seeds
	- Marzipan
	- Digestive biscuits

Guidelines to Control Your Fiber Intake

During the course of a low residue diet, people need to be smart and follow certain guidelines. These guidelines are provided to help people choose foods that are low in fiber content and do not leave residue. Use these guidelines as high level principles while following a low residue diet.

Let's take a look at these guidelines.

- Buy and use white cereals such as rice based cereals and cornflakes.

- Buy and use cereal products prepared without seeds and nuts.

- Buy and use white or refined bread without nuts, seeds and grains.

- Buy and use white varieties of pasta and rice.

- Buy and use plain white biscuits such as malted milks, rich tea and custard creams.

- Buy and use white varieties scones and crumpets.

- You must always cook the vegetables well from the allowed foods list. Please refer to Stage 3 for the list of allowed vegetables.

- You can use herbs and spices that are ground finely.

- People who have ostomy must avoid highly seasoned food and especially garlic cloves.

- Garlic powder can be consumed in moderation.

- Remove the skin of potatoes before using.

- If you bake at home, always use white flour.

- Try not to consume vegetables and fruits with skins, pips and seeds as they are high in fiber and leaves residue.

- You may try to boil and puree fruits and vegetables. If they don't suit you, stop eating them.

- Always make sure the soups, sauces and meals that you buy from the stores do not have added fruits, vegetables, seeds and nuts in them.

- During the course of low residue diet, you will be restricting a lot of fruits and vegetables which may lead to vitamin C deficiency. Make sure you include and drink a vitamin C rich fresh fruit juice (without bits) or squash every day.

- Do not eat more than 3 servings of fruits per day from the allowed list of fruits provided in Stage 3.

- Always use ground, well cooked or tender poultry, fish, lamb, pork, ham, veal, beef and eggs.

- Do not eat fried and tough, fibrous meats with gristle.

- Avoid highly seasoned sausages and cold cut meats, also known as luncheon meats.

- You may consume tea, coffee and fruit punch in moderation.

- It is recommended that a standard multivitamin with minerals is taken daily. You can check with your doctor or certified dietician on this.

- You can eat deserts and sweets without fruits and nuts.

Stage 4: The High Fiber Diet

This is the final stage where the diverticulitis condition has almost healed and the patient is on his track of adopting a normal eating lifestyle. Though the diverticulitis condition has healed, it is still important that the patient monitors his diet for days to come. This will eliminate any possibility of reoccurrence of the disease.

Goals

Goals of a high fiber diet are to bring back a patient in his normal and healthy eating routine. It aims at enabling the patient to resume his daily life post treatment of diverticulitis. The fiber intake is advised to be monitored carefully so as to not overburden the intestine all of a sudden. Only when a low residue diet shows positive results, does a patient shift to a high fiber diet.

Guidelines for High Fiber Diet

- High fiber diet should be started only after the body adapts to fiber intake through low residue diet.

- High fiber diets should be well complemented by intake of water and other fluids. The water makes absorption of fiber easier and hence aids digestion.

- The fibrous intake should be controlled in portion size. Just because the patient is allowed to take up increased amount of foods, does not mean the portion size does not matter. High fiber diets should be well calculated in portions and only about

25-30 grams of fiber should be eaten on daily basis. Anything more than this will again cause problems of constipation and poor digestion.

- Since most of the diverticulitis condition is cured by this stage, it is quite likely that a patient will fall back to his previous eating habits. It is strongly advised that patients keep off anything that got them to have the disease in first place.

Foods to Include & Exclude in High Fiber Diet

Breads and Starches

High fiber diets may include finely grounded whole grains like wheat, barley etc. Pastas, noodles and rice can be eaten normally as well starches from potatoes, wheat, graham and rye can be included in the diet. It is still desirable to keep off refined flours that may cause indigestion.

Meat and Protein

Soft tender meats like fish and slightly stiffer meats like chicken, eggs, proteins in the form of lentils, cheese particularly cottage cheese are advised to be eaten regularly. Red meat is to be avoided at all costs since it is very high in fat and causes severe indigestion.

Vegetables

All vegetables can be included in the diet especially the green leafy ones that have adequate fiber. However, avoid gas inducing vegetables like cauliflower, broccoli, cabbage, radish and kale.

Fruits

A high fiber diet may include all fruits like apple, oranges, peaches, pears, grapes, watermelon, melon and papaya. Almost all fruits work pretty well since there is no restriction on fiber intake. Dried fruits, whether cooked or raw still remain an exception.

Dairy Products

Milk and milk products, especially yogurt is very good for cure of diverticulitis. Yogurts blended with fruits are a good way to keep the gut function under control.

Fats

Fats from red meats pose serious issues in a diverticulitis diet. Olive oils are denser forms of oil that again should be avoided until complete recovery. Any other kinds of fat like butter, margarine, cream fat etc. are all fine to be used in a high fiber diverticulitis guide.

Sweets & Deserts

All sweets can be eaten normally with a condition that they are free from nuts and dried fruits. Honey and sugar can be used for sweetness. Candies and fruit jellies are another way to satiate the sweet tooth while recovering from the diverticulitis disease.

Foods to Completely Avoid In Diverticulitis Disease

- Red meats like goat meet, beef, pork etc.

- Nuts and dried fruits that are hard and have course skin

- Gas inducing fruits and vegetables like cauliflower, broccoli, kale etc.

- Pulp of fruits and vegetables with seeds

- Dense oils like olive oil

- Greasy fried and over processed foods

- Sugary drinks and fizz drinks

- Fat laden fast foods

- Heavy beans like kidney beans, chick peas, black eyed beans etc.

- Corn products like popcorns that are hard and need chewing

Fiber Contents of Foods (Including Market Products)

The following shows the common servings of foods with dietary fiber. It is suggested that you should increase your fiber intake by including fiber from all type of foods and sources. It is important to know that foods from dairy and meat and groups are not good sources of fiber. Always remember and understand that foods that are good sources of fiber are also pretty low in fats.

Breads

Foods	Serving Size	Amount of Fiber (gms)
Bagels	1	0.6
Bran Muffis	1	2.5
Cracked wheat bread	1 slice	1.0
Crisp rye bread	2 crackers	2.0
Crisp wheat bread	2 crackers	1.8
French bread	1 slice	0.7
Italian bread	1 slice	0.3
Mixed grain bread	1 slice	0.9
Oatmeal bread	1 slice	0.5
Pita bread	1 piece	0.4
Pumpernickel bread	1 slice	1.0
Raisin bread	1 slice	0.6
White bread	1 slice	0.4
Whole wheat bread	1 slice	1.4

Cereals

Foods	Serving Size	Amount of Fiber (gms)
All-Bran	1/3 cup	8.5
Bran Buds	1/3 cup	7.9
Bran Chex	2/3	4.6
Cheerios	1 1/4 cups	1.1
Corn Bran	2/3 cup	5.4
Corn Flakes	1 1/4 cups	0.3
Cracklin' Bran	1/3 cup	4.3
Crispy Wheats n' Raisins	3/4 cup	1.3
40% Bran	3/4 cup	4.0
Frosted Mini-Wheats	4 biscuits	2.1
Graham Crackos	3/4 cup	1.7
Grape Nuts	1/4 cup	1.4
Heartland Natural Cereal	1/4 cup	1.3
Honey Bran	7/8 cup	3.1
Most	2/3 cup	3.5
Nutri-Grain, barley	3/4 cup	1.7
Nutri-Grain, corn	3/4 cup	1.8
Nutri-Grain, wheat	3/4 cup	1.8
100% Bran	1/2 cup	8.4
100% Natural Cereal	1/4 cup	1.0
Oatmeal, (cooked regular, quick or instant)	3/4 cup	1.6
Raisin Bran	3/4 cup	4.0
Rice Krispies	1 cup	0.1
Shredded Wheat	2/3 cup	2.6
Special K	1 1/3 cup	0.2
Sugar Smacks	3/4 cup	0.4
Tasteeos	1 1/4 cups	1.0

Total	1 cup	2.0
Wheat Chex	2/3 cup	2.1
Wheaties	1 cup	2.0
Wheat n' Raisin Chex	3/4 cup	2.5
Wheat germ	1/4 cup	3.4

Rice & Pasta

Foods	Serving Size	Amount of Fiber (gms)
Macaroni	1 cup	1.0
Rice, brown	1/2 cup	1.0
Rice, polished	1/2 cup	0.2
Spaghetti, regular	1 cup	1.1
Spaghetti, wheat	1 cup	3.9

Vegetables (Raw)

Foods	Serving Size	Amount of Fiber (gms)
Bean sprouts	1/2 cup	1.5
Celery, diced	1/2 cup	1.1
Cucumber	1/2 cup	0.4
Lettuce, sliced	1/2 cup	0.9
Mushrooms, sliced	1/2 cup	0.9
Onions, sliced	1/2 cup	0.9
Peppers, green, sliced	1/2 cup	0.5
Spinach	1 cup	1.2
Tomato	1	1.5

Vegetables (Cooked)

Foods	Serving Size	Amount of Fiber (gms)
Asparagus, cut	1/2 cup	1.0
Beans (string, green)	1/2 cup	1.6
Broccoli	1/2 cup	2.2
Brussel sprouts	1/2 cup	2.3
Cabbage (red, white)	1/2 cup	1.4
Carrots	1/2 cup	2.3
Cauliflwer	1/2 cup	1.1
Corn, canned	1/2 cup	2.9
Kale leaves	1/2 cup	1.4
Parsnip	1/2 cup	2.7
Peas	1/2 cup	3.6
Potato (with skin)	1	2.5
Potato (without skin)	1	1.4
Spinach	1/2 cup	2.1
Squash, summer	1/2 cup	1.4
Sweet potatoes	1/2	1.7
Turnips	1/2	1.6
Zucchini	1/2 cup	1.8

Fruits

Foods	Serving Size	Amount of Fiber (gms)
Apple (with skin)	1	3.5
Apple (without skin)	1	2.7
Apricot	3	1.8
Apricot, dried	5 halves	1.4
Banana	1	2.4
Blueberries	1/2 cup	2.0

Cantaloupe	1/4 melon	1.0
Cherries, sweet	10	1.2
Grapefruit	1/2	1.6
Grapes	20	0.6
Orange	1	2.6
Peach (with skin)	1	1.9
Peach (without skin)	1	1.2
Pear (with skin)	1/2 large	3.1
Pear (without skin)	1/2 large	2.5
Pineapple	1/2 cup	1.1
Plums, damson	5	0.9
Prunes	3	3.0
Raisins	1/4 cup	3.1
Raspberries	1/2 cup	3.1
Strawberries	1 cup	3.0
Watermelon	1 cup	0.4

Juices

Foods	Serving Size	Amount of Fiber (gms)
Apple	1/2 cup	0.4
Grapefruit	1/2 cup	0.5
Grape	1/2 cup	0.6
Orange	1/2 cup	0.5
Papaya	1/2 cup	0.8

Legumes

Foods	Serving Size	Amount of Fiber (gms)
Baked beans/tomato	1/2 cup	8.9

sauce		
Dried beans, cooked	1/2 cup	4.7
Kidney beans, cooked	1/2 cup	7.3
Lentils, cooked	1/2 cup	7.3
Lima beans, cooked	1/2 cup	4.5
Navy beans, cooked	1/2 cup	6.0

Nuts

Foods	Serving Size	Amount of Fiber (gms)
Almonds	10 nuts	1.1
Filberts	10 nuts	0.8
Peanuts	10 nuts	1.4

Thus, we have thoroughly assessed the various kinds of diets to be followed at various stages of diverticulitis treatment. The diets are progressive in nature and one stage leads to another. These diets are not hard to follow and most ingredients can be found in our everyday households. The intake of these foods when combined with exercise and light physical activities will keep diverticulitis under control.

This Page Has Been Left Blank Intentionally.

Chapter 5

Natural Remedies and Supplements to Cure Diverticulitis

Surgeries and proper dosage of antibiotics is sure to treat the patient out of the ailing condition of diverticulitis. While all of this is a very time intensive and costly process, it is quite feasible for patients to undergo treatment through natural remedies and commonly available ingredients. These remedies may again require prolonged periods of time to improve the condition properly, but with regular care, it is well observed that these treatments and remedies instantly bring relief to the patient. More so, the effect of these remedies continues till long periods where it becomes less likely for the disease to reoccur.

Here is an extensive list of natural remedies and supplements which will make it easier for patients to treat themselves off the diverticulitis disease.

A Prolonged Liquid Diet

After the surgery or in cases where diverticulitis is handled through antibiotics, a liquid diet is the best way that will complement the medication and help the wounds to heal rapidly. It is strongly advised that the patient is put on a liquid diet devoid of excess fiber and non-residual matter. The aim of this kind of diet is easy digestion and non-blockage of any kind in the intestinal region.

Though diverticulitis is caused due to inadequate intake of the fiber rich food, initial days post-surgery should be followed only with clear liquid diet. The diet may include plenty of water, ice pops, aerated drinks that clear passage, and different kinds of soups. This renders some rest to the intestine that does not have to work too hard to digest the food and pass it on for excretion. The intestine hence gets enough time to heal and recover to normal functioning.

After the patient stops complaining of any severe pain or discomfort in the abdomen, he can further be elevated to a semi solid diet that may include portions of added fibers and solid foods. Yogurt and steamed vegetables for example with significantly aid the healing process. Higher fiber foods may be incorporated only after a month of proper rest and depends on extent of healing the patient has undergone.

Rest

It is very important for the body to be put to adequate rest for the treatment of diverticulitis. This puts the intestines to the much needed rest and the condition heals faster. A good amount of rest may also negate the need of surgery in cases where the condition has severed beyond acute uncomplicated diverticulitis. The rest indicates keeping the body off movement for a certain number of days until the signs of diverticulitis disease start disappearing.

The movement should be gradually increased and light exercises should be adopted to bring the body in full swing motion. Though the patients may refrain from any kind of strenuous exercises, they should continue doing lighter forms of workouts until the condition later heals. One should make it a point to involve in daily exercises in the routine to reduce the chances of reoccurrence of the disease or even the mildest of its symptoms.

Multivitamins

Post-surgical recovery in diverticulitis is accompanied by intake of extremely liquid diets that may not completely fulfil the need vitamin needs of the body. Hence it is very important to make sure that the deficiency is being made through intake of additional multivitamin. One should carefully opt for the varieties that comprise of naturally grown ingredients that will eventually affect our bodies in a positive way.

The varieties made from food based supplements, is what one should advisably look for. If one takes artificial supplements made of synthetic ingredients, they might just make the medical condition even worse.

Exercise A Lot-Regularly and In Continuation

As discussed above, post-surgical period should be followed by inactivity and later with gradual exercises. But to safeguard oneself from the risks of diverticulosis and later conversions to diverticulitis, one must make sure to stick to a regular workout regime. This will minimize the chances of a person to contract the disease and will keep risks at bay. This is especially true for people experiencing regular irregularities in digestion, bloating, constipation and other gastric problems. Regular exercise will act on the abdomen, making the muscles stronger in the region and resulting is a stronger digestive mechanism.

Probiotic Supplements

There are well-numbered brands of probiotics available in the market known to support the gut function and improve digestion. These come in small dosages that need to be taken regularly as a part of everyday meal. Opt for the varieties that are organic in nature and that are made from naturally available enzymes. These enzymes control the activities and reactions occurring in the intestine and make sure that it works to its full capacity. Any abnormality or imbalance in the bacterial balance of the intestine may cause infection and succeeding inflammation which may again develop the outbreak of diverticulitis. Hence, incorporating probiotics in the diet will keep off diverticulitis and aid digestion on everyday basis.

Use of Colloidal Silver

When one talks of home and natural remedies for the treatment of diverticulitis, colloidal silver emerges as a promising name. It has special properties that make it effective against germs, viruses and bacteria. It is a natural substance that even acts brutally on pathogens. Colloidal silver works even in conditions where the use of excessive antibiotics fails. It is known to soothe the inflammation and aids in faster recovery of the wounds. Colloidal silver should however be administered under careful observation of a natural medicine practitioner. Though it is a home remedy, it is advised to take complete information of dosage frequency.

Thus, we see that the treatment of diverticulitis does not necessarily have to be painful and expensive. With little care and effort, one can bring themselves out of the risk that the disease poses. Talking of all the measures undertaken, diet still plays a major role. The others will simply be instrumental in making the healing faster. The above methods, if adopted early can save a patient from the distress of a surgery.

This Page Has Been Left Blank Intentionally.

Chapter 6

Lifestyle Changes Necessary to Cure Diverticulitis

Recovering from diverticulitis is a slow and steady process. It depends on the nature of the treatment the patient has undergone and his recovery speed. The patient needs to adopt certain lifestyle changes that will help the condition heal faster and will also help in reducing the possibilities of the condition developing again. It is not possible to change ones entire lifestyle in one go. Nor is it possible to make far-fetched changes in the diet overnight. A patient needs to understand that the changes will take some time to fit into one's lifestyle and that these changes have to be thoroughly consistent to achieve full protection from the ailment.

Go On the Rest Mode

There is nothing more crucial than lending much required rest to the body to heal up. Patients should not bother about being in bed all day long. This is what exactly is needed for the condition to become better. This is particularly true for milder forms of diverticulitis which is curable with the help of medications alone. There may arise absolutely no need of painful and cringe worthy operations. Adequate rest would suffice.

Change the Diet

As discussed previously, diet is the major factor to control and cure diverticulitis. In the initial stages, it has to be solely rich in fluids and water. Gradually, it leads to taking in of very less fibrous foods that are easy to digest. The intake of solid food may take some time until the intestines have fully recovered. Solid foods will restrict smooth movement of food in the intestines, causing food to get stuck with its inability to pass out without restriction. The pressure thus applied may cause pouch formation leading to diverticulitis. Patients hence must be headstrong in adopting a whole new diet to cure them-selves faster.

Incorporate Fresh Fruits and Vegetables in the Diet

Diverticulosis results from lack of fiber and coarse grains in the diet. This is particularly true for fat laden diets that provide little or no nutrition to the body. One must have at least three portions of fruits and vegetables in the entire day. The meal platter should also have greater portions of fruits, vegetables and roughage that lend enough fiber to the body to ease out digestions and keep the digestive tract healthy. Fruits and vegetables are also potent in vitamins and other nutrients necessary to help the bodily functions. Hence, a higher intake of fruits and vegetables will add to your overall health and not just for the cure of diverticulitis. The body will see improvement in overall activity and resistances against a wide variety of diseases.

Give Up On Red Meat

Red meat is the hard kind of meat that causes a variety of gastric problems. It is very difficult to digest and throws a lot of pressure on the intestines for grinding and absorption. Hence, it is very difficult to get it out of the system. Some say that red meat is not even fit for human consumption but well it is very much a part of diets around the world. Red meat has blood and high fat content that in any ways not good for human digestive system. The blood in the red meat may contain enzymes and bacteria that may spread infection in the gut thereby leading to digestive ailments that pile up to become diverticulitis. The high fat content again causes low nutrient absorption problems. To cure diverticulitis, it may still be advised to eat softer meats like fish flesh, chicken and other softer meats that are protein rich and provide body with nutrition.

Give Up On Alcohol

It is strongly advised that the patient either completely gives up on alcohol or at least keeps the intake under strict check. Alcohol disturbs the digestive function as much as it affects the liver. The functioning of both is closely linked and one directly affects the other. Bad quality or excessive alcohol may cause bacterial infection in the gut. Regular alcohol intake also causes dehydration that leads to removal of water from the body. If this continues for long periods, it may cause problems of constipation and poor stomach health.

Keep Obesity under Control

Obesity is the cause of major diseases in the human body. Excessive fat in the body makes people lethargic and drives them away from physical activity. The excess fat on the abdominal region also put pressure on the internal organs and cause problems in digestions. People with high obesity usually are observed to have high number of gastric problems. So it is really important to keep obesity under control through a combination of diet and exercise. This will also reflect positively on the other organs of the body and will improve psychological confidence also.

Drink Plenty of Water

It has been rightly said that water is a wonder drug. It is the best medicine to human body, so one should make sure to have plenty of it. When the patient is treated of diverticulitis, it is important to maintain proper fluid levels in the body. Proper fluid levels will aid digestion and smooth removal of excreta from the body. There should also be enough water in the body to ensure proper absorption of nutrients in the body. Approximately 8 glasses of water a day keeps a person hydrated all day long.

Exercise Regularly

Exercising cannot be compromised in any forms for complete treatment of diverticulitis. 30 minute moderate exercise for at least 30 minutes each day will be beneficial in keeping off risks of developing diverticulitis.

Hence, we have seen that there are different lifestyle changes that will ascertain a person's well-being against the diverticulitis disease. People must be proactive and forward in adopting these changes and must not show ignorant behavior during recovery. Such ignorance on the part of the patient can further impair the situation, hence making it difficult to bring it under proper medical control.

Wrapping up!

Diverticulitis is a common lifestyle disease mostly caused due to poor diet intake that is deficient in fiber. It is a digestive ailment that occurs in milder forms to a majority of people. The large intestine is the major area that gets affected by the disease. Most cases can be treated through diet and antibiotics. In case of severity of the disease, surgery needs to be adopted. It is necessary to adopt a healthy lifestyle to minimize the risk of acquiring the disease. A blend of exercises and the high fiber diet is the key to combat diverticulitis.

At last, I would like to thank you for reading this book and hope that you will create a new healthier you!

Made in the USA
Charleston, SC
09 July 2016